Soumia MISSOUM
Ghalia KHELLAF
Mourad LAHMAR

Mastering peritoneal dialysis in six steps

Soumia MISSOUM
Ghalia KHELLAF
Mourad LAHMAR

Mastering peritoneal dialysis in six steps

ScienciaScripts

Imprint

Any brand names and product names mentioned in this book are subject to trademark, brand or patent protection and are trademarks or registered trademarks of their respective holders. The use of brand names, product names, common names, trade names, product descriptions etc. even without a particular marking in this work is in no way to be construed to mean that such names may be regarded as unrestricted in respect of trademark and brand protection legislation and could thus be used by anyone.

Cover image: www.ingimage.com

This book is a translation from the original published under ISBN 978-613-8-42572-4.

Publisher:
Sciencia Scripts
is a trademark of
Dodo Books Indian Ocean Ltd., member of the OmniScriptum S.R.L Publishing group
str. A.Russo 15, of. 61, Chisinau-2068, Republic of Moldova Europe
Printed at: see last page
ISBN: 978-620-4-06656-1

Foreword :

It was love at first sight between me and peritoneal dialysis in my early years in nephrology, a technique that brings together the nephrologist, the resuscitator and the pediatrician with the sole aim of saving human lives.

And after these 14 long years of experience that I have accumulated, I would like to transmit this knowledge acquired in the field to young nephrologists and nephrologists' seeds (my dear residents), so that this technique is not denigrated by its own children.

Since there is no future without a past, here is a brief overview of the tumultuous history of peritoneal dialysis, which was first performed in animals in the late 1800s and became a full-fledged technique for humans in the early 1960s.

Peritoneal access was first achieved by intermittent abdominal puncture, later the development of a permanent access to the peritoneal cavity with the Tenckhoff catheter allowed the emergence of this therapeutic modality in chronic renal failure and subsequently the development of continuous ambulatory peritoneal dialysis and automated peritoneal dialysis.

In Algeria, the treatment of chronic end-stage renal failure started in 1973 in Algiers with haemodialysis and it is only in 1980 that continuous ambulatory peritoneal dialysis was introduced.

Through this manuscript and in six steps, I will guide you to a total mastery of peritoneal dialysis, while hoping that the new generation of nephrologists, resuscitators and pediatricians will promote this valuable technique.

Soumia Missoum
Senior Lecturer "A" in Nephrology

Summary:

LIST OF ABBREVIATIONS

A

AA: amino acids

APEX: accelerated peritoneal equilibration examination ASP: abdomen without preparation

C

Cm H2O: centimetre of water Creat: creatinineemia

Cm: centimetre Cl: clearance

D

D: dialysate

D0: dialysate time 0 DP: peritoneal dialysis

APD: automated peritoneal dialysis

CAPD: chronic ambulatory peritoneal dialysis

F

RF: residual renal function

G

Gr: gram

H

H: time

HD: hemodialysis

I

CKD: chronic renal failure

CKD: end-stage renal disease BMI: body mass index

K

K: potassium Kg: kilogram

L

L: litre

M

M: meter

M2: square meter Meq: milli-equivalent Min: minute

Ml: millilitre Mmol: milli moles

N

Na: sodium

P

P: plasma
PET: peritoneal equilibration test PIP: intraperitoneal pressure PKR: polycystic kidney disease
PNN: poly-nuclear neutrophils

S

SC: body surface area

T

BP: blood pressure

U

U: urine
UF: ultra filtration
IU: International Unit

V

Vol: volume
VIP: intraperitoneal volume

List of figures :

<h1 style="text-align:center"><u>List of tables:</u></h1>

Table I: Main transfers through the peritoneal membrane .

Table II: 2017 International Peritoneal Dialysis Society recommendation for treatment of peritonitis in PD.

Table III: Maximum intraperitoneal volume according to PIP.

Table IV: Influence of stasis time and intraperitoneal volume on dialysis quality.

The principle of peritoneal dialysis is to install a regularly renewed artificial ascites allowing contact between a physiological liquid (dialysate) introduced via a catheter on one side and the patient's blood on the other, through a highly vascularized natural membrane which is the peritoneum. **(Figure 1)**

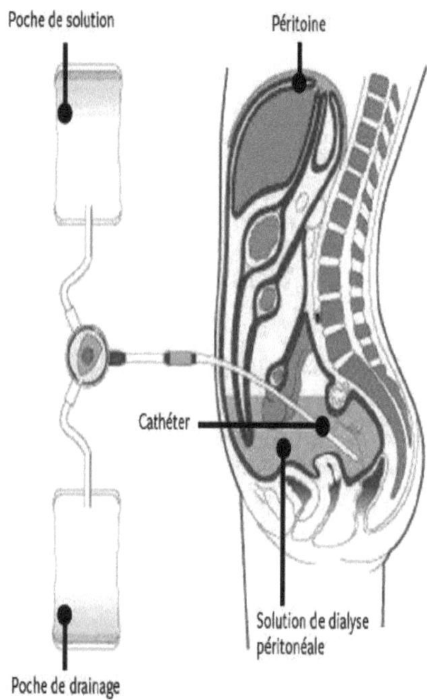

Figure 1: Principles of peritoneal dialysis.

The exchange between dialysate and blood is governed by two processes:

1-   **<u>Diffusion:</u>** the dissolved substances migrate between the blood and the dialysate, according to their concentration gradient until a concentration balance is reached on both sides of the peritoneum. It is therefore logical that the composition of the dialysate is judiciously elaborated in order to allow the drainage of waste products from the blood towards the peritoneal cavity, such as urea, and at the same time a supplementation of certain substances that are deficient in the patient, such as calcium. **(Table I)**

	Plasma	Peritoneal membrane	Peritoneal cavity
Urea (mmol/L)	30	⟶	0
Creatinine (Imol/L)	820	⟶	0
Sodium (mmol/L)	134	⟶	132
Potassium (mmol/L)	5,20	⟶	0
Bicarbonates (mmol/L)	21	⟶	0
Lactates (mmol/L	Inf a 2	⟵	35 à 40
Ionized calcium (mmo1/L)	1,18	⟵	1,25 à 1,75
Phosphorus (mmol/L)	2,10	⟶	0
Uric acid (micromol/L)	460	⟶	0
Glucose (g/L)	1	⟵	10 à 40

Table I: Major transfers across the peritoneal membrane.

2-   **Ultrafiltration:** plasma water is attracted to the peritoneal cavity by an osmotic agent present in the dialysate, generally glucose, the quantity of ultrafiltrated water depends essentially on the concentration of the osmotic agent and its susceptibility to be reabsorbed by the body. Indeed, if we take for example glucose which is the most used osmotically active molecule, its effect will progressively decrease throughout the stasis time, since it is freely absorbed by the peritoneum, hence the decrease of its concentration in the dialysate and a decrease of its ultrafiltration effect, so it is imperative to renew the dialysate. **(Figure 2)**

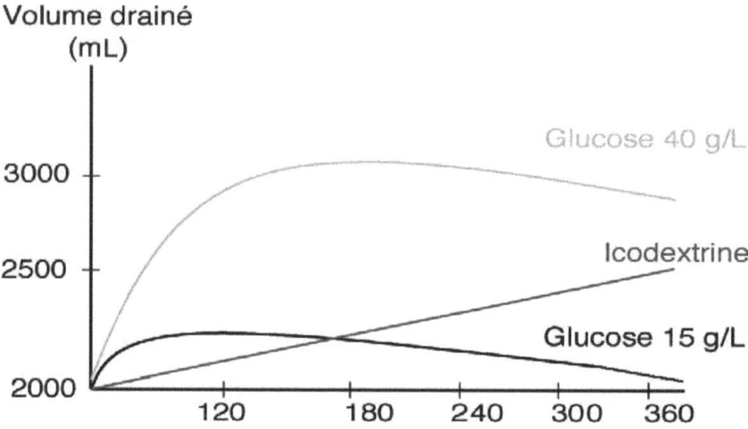

Figure 2: Ultrafiltration according to osmotic agent and stasis time.

II.   RFP Indications:

Peritoneal dialysis offers several advantages to patients, as it is a home treatment, compatible with a social and school life, with less dietary restrictions.

In addition, there are undeniable medical advantages such as better cardiovascular stability, preservation of residual diuresis and vascular capital.

Peritoneal dialysis is above all the choice of the patient, provided that he is clearly informed and supported by his doctor. Nevertheless, this technique is the only one possible in certain circumstances, such as cardiac insufficiency, contraindications to anticoagulation and, of course, exhaustion of the vascular supply.

III.   Contraindications of PD :

The contraindications of PD are more due to clinical situations in which it would be impossible to perform this technique effectively, among these situations:

-        Those which reduce the exchange surface such as a history of major abdominal surgery, or digestive pathologies (stoma, divertivulosis, ascites.....)
-        Those that increase the intraperitoneal pressure and therefore reduce the amount of dialysate that can be infused, such as pregnancy of more than 6 months or significant polycystic kidney disease.

-       Those where the increase in intra-peritoneal pressure induced by PD can cause decompensation of pre-existing pathologies such as in patients suffering from severe respiratory insufficiency (by reduction of the diaphragmatic stroke), or hernias.

-       Those where metabolic complications induced by PD can cause decompensation of pre-existing pathologies such as severe malnutrition or major disorders of carbohydrate-lipid metabolism.

-       Those where the risk of infection is increased: patients with limited hygiene, visually impaired, or homeless.

-       Patients with high purification requirements: obese and anuric patients.

IV.   The six steps to mastering PD :

1.   Unlocking the secrets of the peritoneum

Exchanges take place essentially in the parietal peritoneum, which represents only 10% of the total surface area. During the day, when the patient is standing or sitting, the dialysate is found in the most sloping part of the peritoneal cavity, but in the evening, when the patient lies down, the dialysate spreads out over the entire posterior part of this cavity, thus increasing the exchange surface.

The peritoneum consists of a microvillous unicellular layer called the mesothelium, resting on a basement membrane and separated from the blood capillaries by an interstitial tissue, rich in fibroblasts.

There are three types of pores of different sizes in the endothelium of peritoneal capillaries. (**Figure 3**)

•   The small pores are the seat of the passage of water and molecules of low molecular weight, electrolytes, urea, creatinine, glucose ....ect. 12

•   The ultra small pores or aquaporins, the most numerous, ensure the exclusive transport of free water.

•   The large pores, few in number, allow the passage of large substances, such as proteins, glucose polymers (icodextrin).

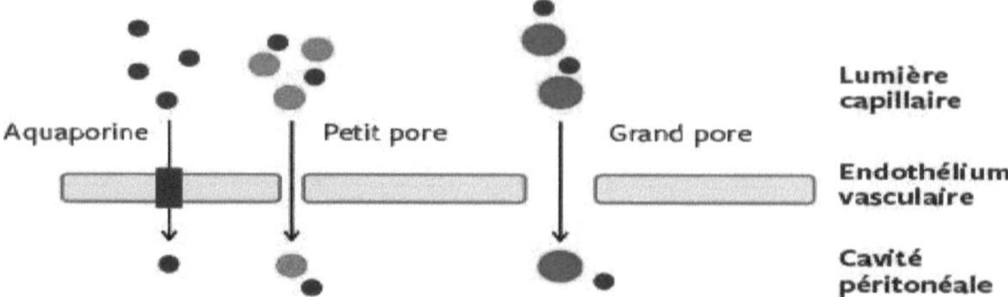

Figure 3: Three-pore model

Each peritoneum is unique, which explains the great variability between patients, in fact the distribution of pores is different between individuals and conditions the nature of the peritoneum either hyper or hypo permeable (more details in the explorations chapter).

2. Become familiar with the material :
a) The peritonealcatheter:

The peritoneal catheter is a permanent catheter, which can remain in place for many years in the absence of complications.

The ideal catheter should ensure a good flow of dialysate during infusion and drainage without leaks and minimize the risk of peritoneal infections.

The most commonly used catheters are the double cuff TENCKHOFF catheters (one internal for fixation to the peritoneum and the other external in the subcutaneous tunnel) and swan neck or straight catheters. (**Figure 4**).

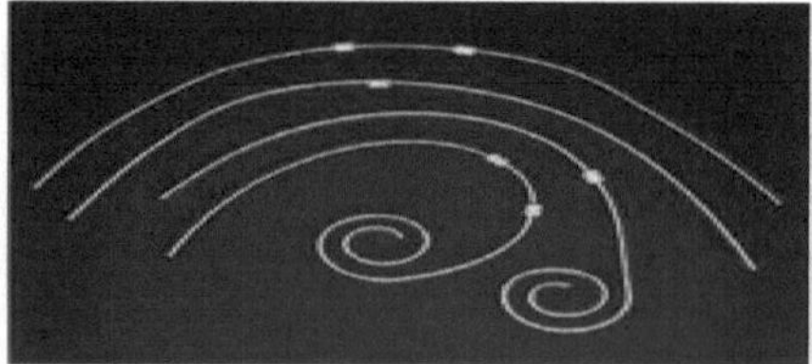

Figure 4: Peritoneal catheter 13

The chronic peritoneal catheter has an intra- and extra-peritoneal portion (**Figure 5**), the latter comprising a subcutaneous part, which allows the catheter to be anchored by the cuff, and an external part beyond the emergence orifice, preferably oriented downwards in adults and children over 3 years of age (subumbilical) in order to allow permanent evacuation of secretions favoured by gravity; for children under 3 years of age, the exit is preferably supraumbilical to avoid contact of the catheter with the diapers.

The internal end of the catheter is placed in the cul-de-sac of Douglas, which is the most sloping part of the cavity, thus allowing optimal drainage. Swan neck catheters are more stable in this position than straight catheters, thus effectively avoiding displacement and malfunction.

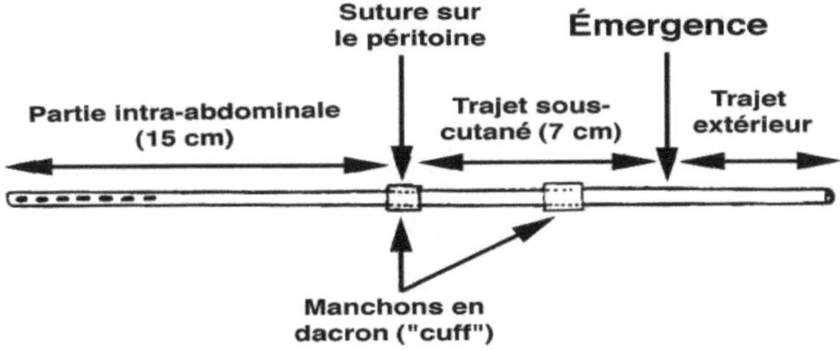

Figure 5: Different parts of the peritoneal catheter.

The choice of the size of the catheter must be adapted to the age and, more precisely, the height of the patient. It corresponds to the estimated distance between the umbilicus and the cul de sac of Douglas, which varies according to the size of the individual, to which is added the length of the subcutaneous path and the external portion of the catheter:

- The newborn: 32 cm.
- The infant: 37 cm.
- Child : 42cm.
- The big child: 57 cm.
- Adult: 62 cm.

An unprepared abdomen must be performed after the catheter has been placed in order to check that the catheter is in place, i.e. in the cul de sac of Douglas.

The Dialysat:

Peritoneal dialysis solutions exist in several concentrations of glucose, packed in transparent plastic bags, with a well studied composition (**Table I**). In Algeria, the PAC is presented with two bags connected by tubules, one filled with 2 liters of dialysate and the other empty allowing the drainage of the intraperitoneal liquid, There are several types of PD bags that differ according to several parameters:

1) the nature of the osmotic agent used :

a.   Glucose
b.   Poly maltose (extraneal)
c.   Amino acids (Nutrineal)

Glucose is not an ideal osmotic agent even if it is the cheapest, since it easily crosses the peritoneum, it is absorbed in the blood and then metabolized by the organism, the degradation products of glucose attack the peritoneum and accelerate its fibrosis.

Icodextrin due to its large size induces water displacement through small pores; this leads to an increase in the clearance of low molecular weight solutes. It increases UF during long periods of stasis up to 12 hours for CAPD (nocturnal stasis), up to 16 hours for DPA (diurnal stasis), therefore it should not be used for short contact times, its efficiency in terms of UF is similar to hypertonic glucose while decreasing the glucose load.

Nutrineal® is a PD solution of 15 amino acids at 1.1%, equivalent to an isotonic solution in terms of ultrafiltration and clearance of small solutes. It has the advantage of offsetting protein losses (4 to 6 g/day of albumin) and can improve nutritional status in malnourished patients and during episodes of peritonitis, however amino acids are not more effective than glucose as an osmotic agent. Nutrineal® should be prescribed at a rate of one bag per day in CAPD, and prescribed at a rate of one bag per night in APD.

2) the concentration of the osmotic agent, in this case glucose:

a.   Isotonic (13g/L)
b.   Intermediate (22.7g/L)
c.   Hypertonic (38.6g/L)

The higher the glucose concentration, the higher the osmotic pressure, which leads to additional fluid removal, but hypertonic solutions are also more aggressive to the peritoneum.

3) the nature of the buffer substance :

a.   Extraneal (Lactate 40 mmol ph : 5.5)

b.   Physioneal (bicarbonate 25 mmol/L lactate 15 mmol/L

The acidic PH of the Extraneal and Glucose bags attacks the peritoneum in the long term, which conditions the survival of the technique. We talk about bio-incompatibility, the more physiological Physioneal solutions are more respectful of the membrane.

There are two types of packaging: the one with one compartment (acid: pH 5.5), which is the only one available in Algeria, and the one with two compartments **(Figure 6- 7)**.

For bi-compartment bags, one contains the alkaline solution of the buffer, the other contains the acidic solution based on glucose and electrolytes, the mixture of the two after being brought into contact makes it possible to obtain the ready-to-use solution. This separation avoids the formation of glucose degradation products during heat sterilization (caramelization) and allows to obtain extemporaneously solutions at physiological pH (pH 7 to 7.4).

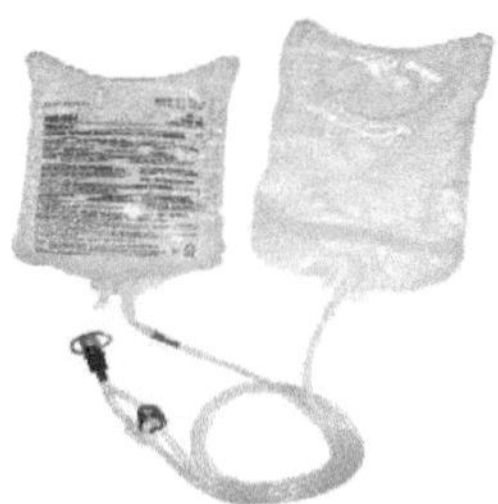

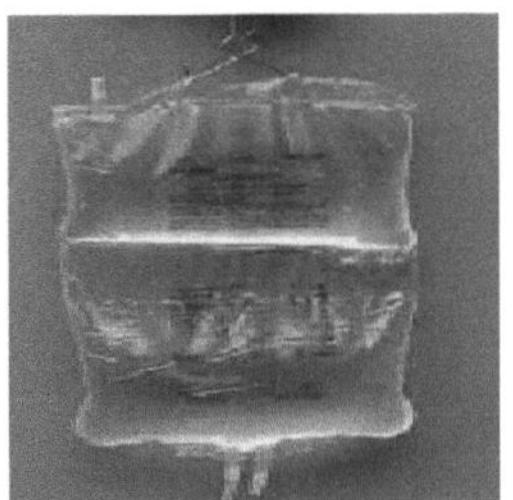

Figure 6: Single compartment system compartment system

Figure   7:   Dual

The choice of dialysate will depend on the resources available but also on the needs of each patient, in terms of ultrafiltration (glucose concentration, Icodextrin), state of malnutrition or inflammation (Nutrineal), preservation of the peritoneal membrane (Physioneal), and the phosphocalcic balance

(fluid calcium concentration 1.25 if PTH low-1.75 mmol/l if PTH high).

b)   Extenders or extension lines:

Represents a tubing that we adapt to the external portion of the catheter allowing us to connect the latter to the PD bags, for each brand of suppliers of dialysate bags there is a specific extender, in Algeria two laboratories exist Baxter and Fresenius. (**Figure 8**)

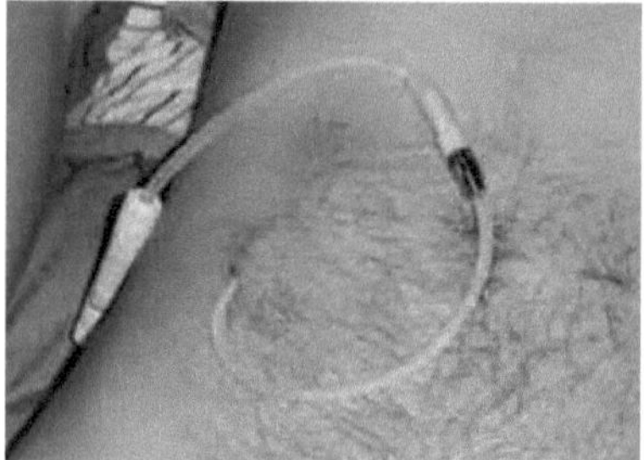

Figure 8: Extender

c)   The caps:

Allows for a sterile and airtight seal at the end of the extension, the cap must be replaced after each use. (**Figure 9**)

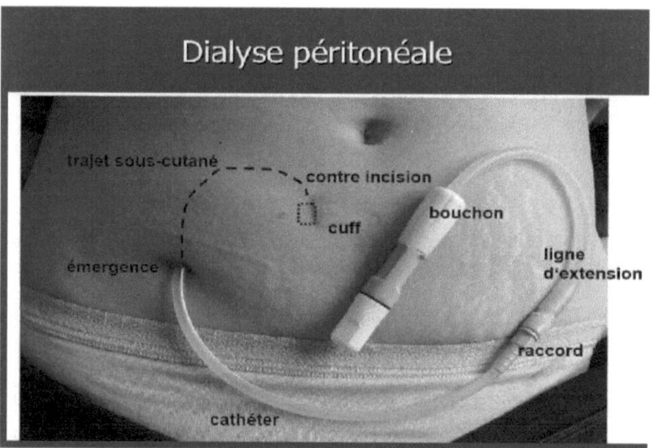

Figure 9: Visible parts of the PD materials

d)   Pocket scales :

This allows us to control the exact amount infused to the patient. (**Figure 10**)

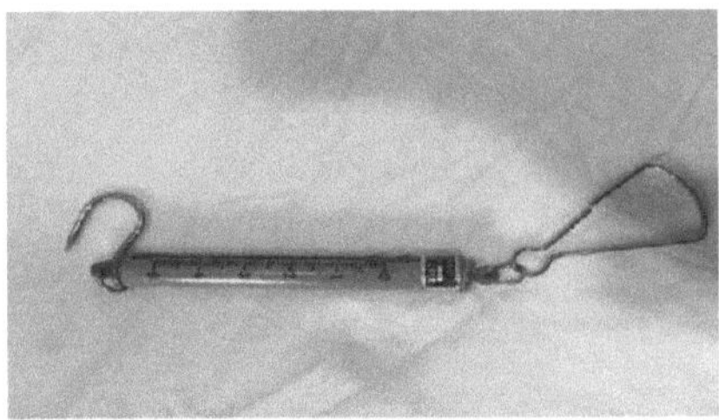

Figure 10: Pocket scale

3. Master the different PD techniques:

a) CAPD (continuous ambulatory peritoneal dialysis): Diurnal and manual the patient is autonomous with a single bag system, it consists of :

- 4 exchanges (3 daytime + 1 nighttime)
- Often at 8H / 12H / 16H /20H
- 7 days a week
- Count 15 to 30 minutes for each manipulation (drainage + infusion).

Each exchange includes **(Figure 11)**:

- Drainage: To drain the peritoneal cavity of the liquid in stasis since the last exchange, the empty bag must be placed in a low position and the clamp that closes the line or the extender must be opened; by gravity, the dialysate must flow from the abdominal cavity to the empty bag.
- Infusion: The new dialysate bag is hung at a high point, which allows it to be emptied by gravity into the peritoneal cavity after opening the line clamp or the extension.
- Stasis: This is the period during which the dialysis fluid remains in place in the peritoneal cavity. This period is important because exchanges take place.

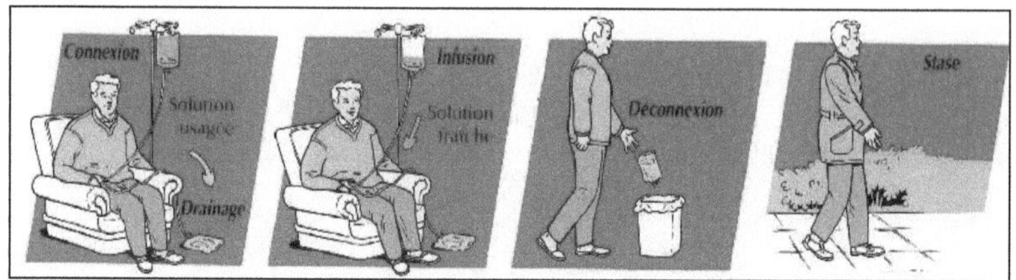

Figure 11: Process of a CAPD exchange

b)   APD (automated peritoneal dialysis):

The use of a machine allows for the delivery of larger quantities of dialysate while automatically ensuring exchanges, so it is possible to use a device to increase the efficiency of PD and to help the patient to perform exchanges.

The device or cycler (**Figure 12**), is a machine that automatically manages exchanges according to a pre-established program, it is an equipment suitable for home treatment.

The patient connects his extension cord to the device, which is equipped with a sufficient number of bags for the entire session, i.e. 15 to 25 L.

The cycler takes care of all the stages of dialysis: drainage, heating, infusion. The machine distributes the cycles during the patient's sleep, calculates the quantities of solution injected and then of dialysate drained, synchronizes the exchanges and controls the progress of the treatment; the dialysis session lasts 8 to 12 hours.

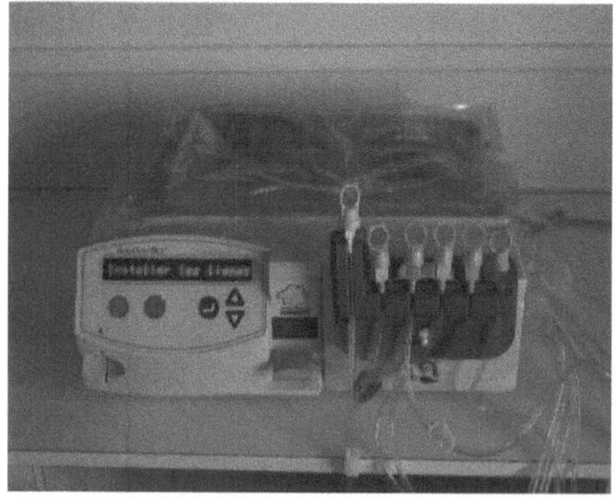

Figure 12: Cycler.

There are several options in CCA:

- Intermittent DPA consists of several cycles in the evening provided by the cycler, with an empty stomach in the morning.
- Continuous cyclic DPA consists of several cycles in the evening provided by the cycler, with a full belly in the morning resulting in a long daytime stasis.
- Optimized cyclic continuous DPA consists of several cycles in the evening provided by the cycler, with a full belly in the morning resulting in a long daytime stasis to which is added a short manual daytime cycle.

4. Integrate the rules of the first prescription:

The rule is to always start with CAPD, even if the patient is planning to undergo APD, in order to check the functioning of the catheter, to familiarize the patient and his entourage with this type of dialysis and above all to keep in mind that patients undergoing APD who complicate a peritonitis will automatically be switched to CAPD in order to receive the continuous intraperitoneal treatment, so all patients undergoing PD must master CAPD.

Ideally, the first prescription is :

- in the case where the function
The residual renal volume is present in 3 exchanges per day of 2 litres for the adult and 30 ml/kg for the child, the first one at 8 a.m. with a glucose-based dialysate and a 4-hour stasis, the second one at noon with an amino acid-based dialysate and an 8-hour stasis, and the last one at 8 p.m. with an icodextrin-based dialysate and a long 12-hour stasis
- in the case where the function
Residual renal function is absent in 4 exchanges per day of 2 liters for the adult and 30 ml/kg for the child, the first one at 08 h with a glucose-based dialysate and a 4h stasis, the second one at noon with an amino acid-based dialysate and a 4h stasis, the third one at 16 h with a glucose-based dialysate and a 4h stasis, and the last one at 20 h with an icodextrin-based dialysate and a long 12 h stasis.

This first prescription will be modified on a case by case basis after evaluation on the 15th day by PD tests (see chapter on dialysis quality).

In Algeria, because of the lack of Nutrineal, the first prescription contains only glucose bags and Icodextrin, with a scheme of 04 exchanges per day (03 diurnal with isotonic glucose bags and one nightly exchange with icodextrin).

5.   Know how to detect and treat complications:

Complications can be early, occurring within 4 weeks after implantation, or late, occurring 4 weeks after.

Early complications are often related to the location of the catheter, while late complications are related to multiple factors other than the surgical procedure.

a)   Mechanical Complications:

i.   Related either to the malfunction of the peritoneal catheter, or to the increase in intraperitoneal pressure.

They may be related to increased intraperitoneal pressure as :

Hernias: Any hernia in the abdominal wall should be surgically corrected before starting peritoneal dialysis treatment. Indeed, hernias will worsen due to the increase in intraperitoneal pressure caused by the presence of dialysate in the cavity. The hernias most frequently encountered after peritoneal dialysis treatment are incisional, umbilical or inguinal. A surgical opinion is essential with a view to surgical reduction of the hernia.

Dialysate leakage: This complication can appear early after a too rapid start of PD or later caused by traction on the catheter or an increase in intraperitoneal pressure. A 10 day interruption is recommended, a slow and progressive resumption of PD with a quantity of infused dialysate reduced to 50 ml/kg per exchange is the rule. The quantity should be increased very carefully according to the clinic.

Incarceration of the omentum: an extremely painful complication, especially at the time of drainage with a blood-tinged liquid, it corresponds to a

incarceration of the omentum in the holes of the catheter with risk of necrosis, first try a forced infusion in the hope of freeing the omentum if not a replacement of the catheter is necessary.

ii.   Related to peritoneal catheter dysfunction:

-     **Drainage not possible :**

Drainage failure (unidirectional obstruction) is the most frequently encountered problem and is characterized by the inability to empty the peritoneal cavity. The causes of this complication may be the presence of blood or fibrin debris in the lumen of the catheter, rolling of the catheter by the intestinal coils filled with material in case of constipation, or displacement of the proximal end of the catheter out of the pelvis.

- **Injection not possible :**

The impossibility of injecting is due either to a kink in the catheter, often in its subcutaneous course, or to the presence of debris in its lumen.

Treatment of catheter malfunction includes: changing the body position at the time of exchanges (lying on the side, squatting, etc.), a laxative in case of constipation, rinsing the catheter with a heparinized solution of isotonic saline. If these manoeuvres fail, it is then possible to try injecting fibrinolytic agents into the catheter and leaving them to act for 1 hour, and if necessary replacing the catheter.

b)   Infectious complications:
i.   Infections of the orifice:

It is defined by the presence of a purulent discharge; and may be suspected in the presence of peri-orificial redness, swelling or pain.
The isolation of a germ associated with the presence of pus requires local care and local antibiotic therapy (pyostacin), for 10 to 15 days, in the absence of early treatment there is a great risk of extension to tunnelitis or even peritonitis.

ii.   Tunnelite :

Corresponds to a real abscess located between the two catheter sleeves.
Requiring a 15-day general antibiotic treatment, adapted to the germ isolated by swabbing.

iii.   Peritonitis :

Peritonitis is secondary to the introduction of germs into the dialysate, secondary to an error in handling, infection of the emergence, poor hygiene, or by digestive contingency, the hematological origin is much rarer.

Any turbid drainage fluid should be considered a priori as peritonitis, to be confirmed by a cytology of the dialysate (more than 100 cells/mm3 including at least 50% neutrophils) and culture of the fluid. A double antibiotic therapy according to the antibiogram must be instituted (**Table II**), one generally aims for the probabilistic treatment while waiting for the culture the staphylococcus epidermidis (cephalosporin 1st generation + aminoside) by intra peritoneal way for a duration of 7 to 21 days to which one adds heparin sodium 2500 UI / bag during the first 48 H to avoid the formation of clots of fibrin. The evolution is marked by a clinical response in 24 hours, bacteriological response in 3 days, and the disappearance of leukocytes in 7 days.

Repeated peritonitis exposes the risk of adhesions and permanent alteration of the membrane, which may prevent the technique from being continued.

Three types of peritonitis are to be highlighted:
1-   Mushroom peritonitis is difficult to diagnose (long cultures in specific media) and especially difficult to sterilize even with the new generation of antimycotics.
2-   Fecal peritonitis, a major emergency in PD, requires peritoneal cleansing and a definitive end to the technique.
3-   Chronic sclerosing and encapsulating peritonitis:
It is a rare but serious complication. It is a diffuse peritoneal fibrosis which involves the formation of a neo-membrane tightly surrounding the intestinal ansae and enclosing them in a fibrous gangue forming a cocoon. Clinically, it can occur with sub-occlusive episodes, chronic inflammation and malnutrition. It can appear in PD patients switched to hemodialysis or renal transplantation, especially those put on cyclosporine. Treatment involves stopping PD and transferring to HD, low-dose corticosteroid therapy would reduce adhesions and facilitate surgery, but the prognosis remains poor.

	Intermittent (1 exchange daily)	Continuous (all exchanges)
Aminoglycosides		
Amikacin	2 mg/kg daily (252)	LD 25 mg/L, MD 12 mg/L (253)
Gentamicin	0.6 mg/kg daily (254)	LD 8 mg/L, MD 4 mg/L (255,256)
Netilmicin	0.6 mg/kg daily (233)	MD 10 mg/L (257)
Tobramycin	0.6 mg/kg daily (253)	LD 3 mg/kg, MD 0.3 mg/kg (258,259)
Cephalosporins		
Cefazolin	15–20 mg/kg daily (260,261)	LD 500 mg/L, MD 125 mg/L (254)
Cefepime	1,000 mg daily (262,263)	LD 250–500 mg/L, MD 100–125 mg/L (262,263)
Cefoperazone	no data	LD 500 mg/L, MD 62.5–125 mg/L (264,265)
Cefotaxime	500–1,000 mg daily (266)	no data
Ceftazidime	1,000–1,500 mg daily (267,268)	LD 500 mg/L, MD 125 mg/L (236)
Ceftriaxone	1,000 mg daily (269)	no data
Penicillins		
Penicillin G	no data	LD 50,000 unit/L, MD 25,000 unit/L (270)
Amoxicillin	no data	MD 150 mg/L (271)
Ampicillin	no data	MD 125 mg/L (272,273)
Ampicillin/Sulbactam	2 gm/1 gm every 12 hours (274)	LD 750–100 mg/L, MD 100 mg/L (253)
Piperacillin/Tazobactam	no data	LD 4 gm/0.5 gm, MD 1 gm/0.125 gm (275)
Others		
Aztreonam	2 gm daily (242)	LD 1,000 mg/L, MD 250 mg/L (243,244)
Ciprofloxacin	no data	MD 50 mg/L (276)
Clindamycin	no data	MD 600 mg/bag (277)
Daptomycin	no data	LD 100 mg/L, MD 20 mg/L (278)
Imipenem/Cilastatin	500 mg in alternate exchange (244)	LD 250 mg/L, MD 50 mg/L (236)
Ofloxacin	no data	LD 200 mg, MD 25 mg/L (279)
Polymyxin B	no data	MD 300,000 unit (30 mg)/bag (280)
Quinupristin/Dalfopristin	25 mg/L in alternate exchange[a] (281)	no data
Meropenem	1 gm daily (282)	no data
Teicoplanin	15 mg/kg every 5 days (283)	LD 400 mg/bag, MD 20 mg/bag (229)
Vancomycin	15–30 mg/kg every 5–7 days[b] (284)	LD 30 mg/kg, MD 1.5 mg/kg/bag (285)
Antifungals		
Fluconazole	IP 200 mg every 24 to 48 hours (286)	no data
Voriconazole	IP 2.5 mg/kg daily (287)	no data

LD = loading dose in mg; MD = maintenance dose in mg; IP = intraperitoneal; APD = automated peritoneal dialysis.

[a] Given in conjunction with 500 mg intravenous twice daily (281).

[b] Supplemental doses may be needed for APD patients.

Table II: 2017 International Society of Peroneal Dialysis

peri

toneal dialysis for the treatment of peritonitis in PD.

c) Complications related to alterations in peritoneal membrane :

i.   Loss of ultrafiltration :

The loss of ultrafiltration (UF) is the main consequence of morphological alterations of the peritoneum due to infectious aggressions and glucose degradation products. It compromises the balance of both water and sodium balances and increases morbidity and mortality, particularly in the cardiovascular system.

ii.   Hemoperitoneum :

A small amount of hemoperitoneum is very common in the hours following peritoneal catheter implantation and usually appears within 24 to 48 hours.

No particular treatment is necessary, but if the haemoperitoneum persists or worsens, we may suspect injury to a vessel in the wall or to a viscera which may have occurred during the manoeuvres for introducing the catheter.

iii.   Pneumoperitoneum :

The presence of small quantities of air in the peritoneum is a fairly frequent occurrence, the pneumoperitoneum is generally asymptomatic, the origin of the air is most often external. In this case no particular treatment needs to be applied, but the situation is quite different when the origin of the pneumoperitoneum is endogenous due to a perforation of a hollow organ (digestive tract), in which case the surgical treatment appropriate to intestinal perforation is applied.

d)   Metabolic complications:

The daily glucose load in the dialysate, especially in hypertonic bags, is frequently responsible for hyper triglyceridemia, obesity, hyper insulinism and glucose intolerance or diabetes mellitus.

Lipoprotein disturbances have been reported, including a decrease in HDL-cholesterol and a consequent increase in the risk of atheroma.

During PD there is a protein loss (5-15 gr per day) increased by the episodes of peritonitis, a sufficient protein intake (1.2-1.5 gr/kg/day) associated with Nutrineal bags is necessary to avoid undernutrition.

6.   How to judge a peritoneum :

Each peritoneum has its own characteristics, in terms of ultrafiltration and purification, which strongly influence the medical prescription.

The study of peritoneal permeability is based on two tests

- **The PET (Peritoneal Equilibration Test):**

According to Twardowski, is performed using 2 L of semi-hypertonic solution (glucose 25 g/L) over a four-hour period. It is imperative to use the same solution during the long overnight stasis preceding the test. The ratios between the concentration in the dialysate and that in the plasma (D/P) of substances appearing in the peritoneal cavity (urea, creatinine, phosphorus), and those disappearing (D/Do) such as glucose, at time 0 (start of dialysis), at the second hour and at the fourth hour are studied. Four types of peritoneal permeability can thus be distinguished, ranging from frank or moderate hypopermeability to moderate or frank hyperpermeability **(Figure 13)**.

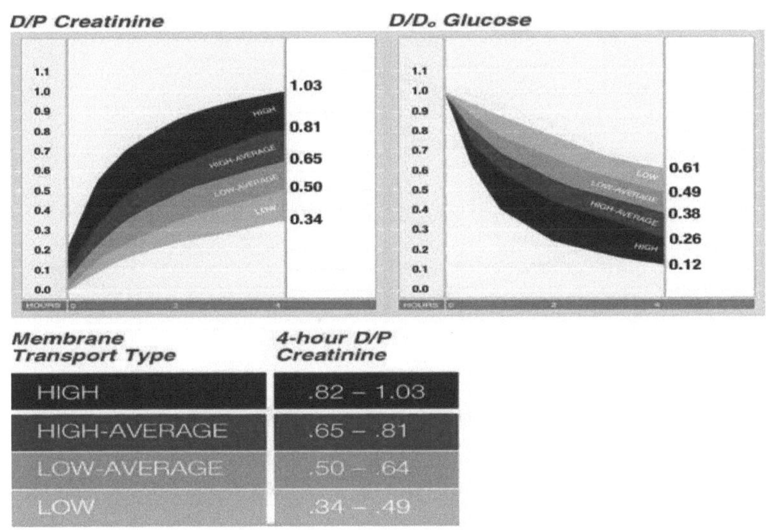

Membrane Transport Type	4-hour D/P Creatinine
HIGH	.82 – 1.03
HIGH-AVERAGE	.65 – .81
LOW-AVERAGE	.50 – .64
LOW	.34 – .49

-        **The APEX: accelerated peritoneal equilibration examination**
According to Verger, also appreciates the net ultrafiltration and the sieving of sodium, witness of the free water transfer, it is carried out with a hypertonic solution (glucose 40 g/L) over a period of two hours.

The APEX curves of urea crossed with the glucose decay curve is the reference, expressed in percentages, the curves cross at a given time or APEX time (normal 65 ± 30 minutes).

The APEX time is increased in case of hypopermeability, decreased in case of hyperpermeability (**Figure 14**).

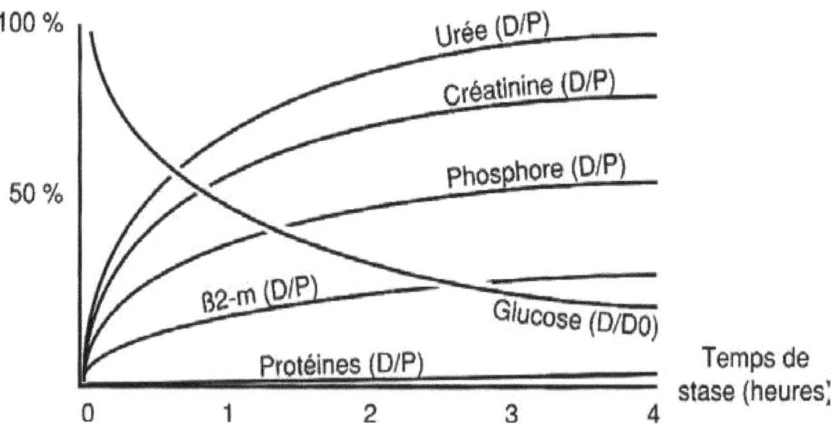

Figure 14: APEX test

In total :

Hypo permeable peritoneum has a poor purifying power, but at the same time thanks to this hypo permeability there is very little absorption of glucose hence a maintenance of the osmotic gradient and a good ultrafiltration through the aquaporins. For these patients it is imperative to maximize the quality of dialysis by proposing long stasis, if they are anuric the Switch to hemodialysis is necessary.

Hyperpermeable peritones have an excellent purifying power, but at the same time this hyperpermeability generates an important and fast glucose release, which leads to a decrease of the osmotic gradient and a fast loss of ultrafiltration. For these patients it is imperative to maximize the quality of dialysis by proposing short stases, they are excellent candidates for APD.

V.   Quality of dialysis:

In addition to the prescription, the quality of the dialysis depends on two factors:

1- the quality of the peritoneum (see corresponding chapter).

2- The quantity of dialysate tolerated by the patient: determined thanks to the intra-peritoneal pressure It is used to assess the tolerance to the intra-peritoneal volume and thus constitutes an aid to prescribe the infusion volume. The principle is the same as for the peripheral venous pressure, based on the measurement of the height of the dialysate rising in the drainage line which forms a right angle from the middle axillary line to the stem (the drainage bag being fixed upwards), for a given volume of intraperitoneal dialysate (**Figure 15**).

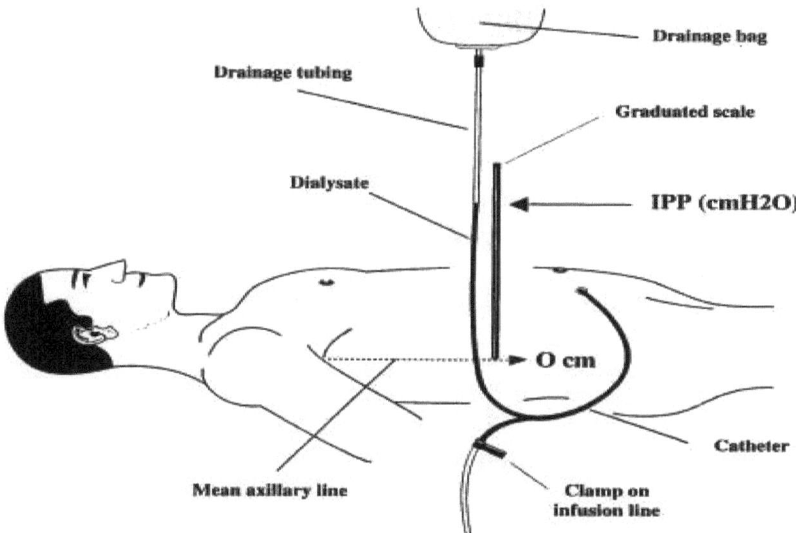

Figure 15: Intraperitoneal pressure test

The normal I.P.P. of an adult is 12 +/- 2cm H2O for an intra-peritoneal volume of 2 litres.

The I.P.P. increases linearly by 2cm H2O per additional intraperitoneal liter (**Table III**).

An I.P.P. value < 18cm H2O corresponds to an intra-peritoneal volume that is generally well tolerated for a patient without cardiac or respiratory insufficiency.

An I.P.P. value > 18cm H2O is often poorly tolerated clinically (sleep disorders, nausea, vomiting, polypnoea, abdominal pain).

The use of dialytic volumes that give a sub-standard I.P.P. ensures optimal ultrafiltration and minimizes lymphatic reabsorption.

I.P.P. measured with an intraperitoneal volume of 2 litres	Maximum volume to be prescribed
< 14 cm H2O	3 litres
15 cm H2O	2.5 litres
16 cm H2O	2 litres
17 cm H2O	1.5 litres
18 cm H2O	1 litre

Table III: Maximum intraperitoneal volume according to PIP

To evaluate the quality of peritoneal dialysis, the dialysis dose must be calculated
This makes it possible to affirm that dialysis is "adequate", i.e. that it corresponds to a minimal dose of dialysis with a favourable influence on morbimortality.

And for this, three parameters must be evaluated
a)   **Residual renal function:**
Plays a major role, it corresponds to the glomerular filtration rate evaluated by the sum of the weekly renal clearances of urea and creatinine, divided by 2. knowing that :

VI.   Weekly renal creatinine clearance=
(Urine creatinine/blood creatinine) x diuresis in litres x 7.

VII.   Weekly renal urea clearances=
(Urine urea/blood urea) x diuresis in litres x 7.
It is maintained longer in peritoneal dialysis than in hemodialysis. It determines

the peritoneal dialysis modality, with a preferential prescription of DPA if the FRR is reduced (<2 ml/minute).

b)   Total creatinine clearance:

Obtained by summing renal and peritoneal creatinine clearance.

It requires a strict collection of urine and all the dialysate drained over 24 hours, and is expressed in litres per week and per 1.73 m2 of body surface.

Weekly total creatinine clearance = renal + peritoneal creatinine clearance. Knowing that :

VIII.   Weekly peritoneal creatinine clearance =

(24 h dialysate creatinine / blood creatinine) x 24 hour drained volume in litres x 7.

The result obtained from the weekly total creatinine clearance must be reported at 1.73 m2 (i.e. the result x 1.73 / body surface area).

c)   The KT/V of urea:

Represents the ratio of the sum of weekly renal and peritoneal urea clearance to the total body water volume expressed in litres. The latter can be estimated from various formulas, including Watson's, taking into account age, height and body weight, but is often equated to 58% of body weight.

(Urea in 24 h dialysate + Urea in 24 h urine) / Blood urea x 7, reported at 58% (therefore the result x 58 / 100).

IX.   Proper dialysis:

It is recommended that the performance of the peritoneal membrane and the criteria for adequate dialysis be assessed one month after the start of treatment and then every 6 to 12 months, unless complications arise.

Adaptation of the dialysis dose takes into account the patient's clinical condition, residual renal function and the need to achieve the defined targets (**Table IV**).

	ULTRAFILTRATION	DIALYTIC TREATMENT
Short contact time	maintenance of the osmotic gradient	decrease of the diffusion time
Contact time Long	loss of osmotic gradient	increase of the diffusion time
Low Intraperitoneal Volume	decrease in glucose load Low PIP	decrease of the volume of diffusion
Large Intraperitoneal Volume	↑ increased glucose load High PIP ↓	↑ increase in the volume of distribution

Table VI: Influence of stasis time and intraperitoneal volume on dialysis quality

The weekly KT/V of urea must be greater than 2.0 in CAPD and 2.2 in APD,

total weekly creatinine clearance must be greater than 60 L/week per 1.73 m2 of body surface area.

KT/V urea is preferable in cases of residual renal function, whereas total creatinine clearance is more reliable in anuric subjects.

The peritoneal dialysis program is adapted according to the degree of peritoneal permeability:

- In case of hyperpermeability, short cycles in DPA are recommended.
- In case of hypopermeability, long cycles of DPCA are prescribed.

However, if the RIF is less than 2 ml/minute in a patient with a body surface area greater than 2 m2, only transfer to hemodialysis can achieve adequate dialysis.

V.　Particularities of peritoneal dialysis in children :

Peritoneal dialysis is the easiest extrarenal dialysis technique to implement in the pediatric population, even in very young children.

Nevertheless some particularities are to be taken with considerations:

-        Peritoneum:
The total surface area of the peritoneum is globally proportional to the weight and size of the subject, and is estimated at 383 to 450 cm²/kg of body weight in children, twice that of adults: 177 to 284 cm/kg, which makes children excellent candidates for PD.
The peritoneum in children is hyperpermeable.

-        Catheter:
The choice of the peritoneal catheter must respond to the variable needs of the children, their age, their autonomy (cleanliness, walking) and the associated disabilities.

The Tenckhoff type peritoneal catheter is the most commonly used in pediatrics. It is available with one or two cuffs and a variable intraperitoneal length of 6.2 to 15 cm. The intra-abdominal end is preferably coiled.

The size of the catheter depends on age:
- In newborns: 32 cm
- In infants: 37 cm
- In children: 42 cm
- For the older child: 57 cm

-        Surgical technique :
The insertion is surgical, from a cutaneous entry orifice, located supra-umbilical with a positioning of the intraperitoneal end of the catheter in the cul-de-sac of Douglas, but para-medial.

The cutaneous exit of the catheter is influenced by the acquisition of cleanliness, as long as the child is wearing nappies, the exit of the catheter is in a lateral or cranial direction, but in case of acquired cleanliness the direction is caudal, avoiding the folded areas.

The catheter is preferably placed on the left, in order to leave the right iliac fossa free for a renal graft, and to benefit from the descending peristalsis of the left colon, which favours the maintenance of the catheter at the bottom of the peritoneal cavity.

- Volume of intraperitoneal dialysate :
The prescription of VIP in pediatrics remains relatively empirical 30 to 50 ml/kg or 600 to 1200 ml/m².

The prescribed volume is lower in infants and newborns than in older children, and is lower in the standing position (CAPD) than in the supine position (APD).

An adaptation time is necessary for the tolerance of a VIP, its increase must be progressive, especially in the postoperative period.

Excess volume is a morbidity factor causing pain, dyspnea, hydrothorax, hernia, vaginal hydrocele, gastroesophageal reflux with anorexia, and loss of ultrafiltration due to lymphatic drainage.

- Complications:

The frequency of hernias is high, especially in small boys, (peritoneovaginal orifice: scrotal hernia or hydrocele). Ligation of the peritoneo-vaginal canal is often necessary.

- Techniques used :

DPA with a cycler and nocturnal session is the most frequently prescribed modality, to preserve schooling but also because the peritoneum in children is of the hyperpermeable type requiring short stasis times and numerous exchanges, this is facilitated by the automated DPA technique.

PD allows the child's abdomen to be prepared to receive a graft, thus maximizing the child's exchange rate by reducing the waiting time.

X.   Conclusion:

Peritoneal dialysis is a tailor-made purification technique, adapted and personalised according to the needs of each patient, nevertheless it requires a rigorous follow-up by an experienced nephrologist.

I finish this manuscript that I hope will help you to tame peritoneal dialysis with a sentence that my master Pr Rayane Tahar used to say to me and that echoed in my heart: "**Peritoneal dialysis is a second choice technique intended for third choice patients and practiced by first choice nephrologists.**

References:

1- Schellartz I, Mettang S, Shukri A, Scholten N, Pfaff H, Early Referral to Nephrological Care and the Uptake of Peritoneal Dialysis. An Analysis of German Claims Data Int J Environ Res Public Health. August 7, 2021

2- Balafa O, Duni A, Tseke P, Rapsomanikis K, Pavlakou P, Ikonomou M, Tatsis V, Dounousi E. Survival of Peritoneal Membrane Function on Biocompatible Dialysis Solutions in a Peritoneal Dialysis Cohort Assessed by a Novel Test J Clin Med. 2021 Aug 18

3- Sachar M, Shah A. Epidemiology, Management, and Prevention of Exit Site Infections in Peritoneal Dialysis Patients. Ther Apher Dial. 2021 Aug 26.

4- Sachdeva B, Zulfiqar H, Aeddula NR. Peritoneal Dialysis 2021 Aug 13. In: StatPearls

5- Mettang T. Lebeaux, D. and M. Touam, *[Peritoneal dialysis-related infections]*. Rev Prat, 2014.

6- Teixido-Planas, J., et al, *Measuring peritoneal absorption with the prolonged peritoneal equilibration test from 4 to 8 hours using various glucose concentrations*. Perit Dial Int, 2014.

7- Sikorska, D., et al, *The importance of residual renal function in peritoneal dialysis*. Int Urol Nephrol, 2016.

8- Wang, L. and T. Wang, *Adequacy of peritoneal dialysis: Kt/V revisited*. Eur Rev Med Pharmacol Sci, 2015.

9-   Borzych-Duzalka, D., et al, *Peritoneal Dialysis Access Revision in Children: Causes, Interventions, and Outcomes.* Clin J Am Soc Nephrol, 2017.

10-   Lebeaux, D. and M. Touam, *[Peritoneal dialysis- related infections].* Rev Prat, 2014

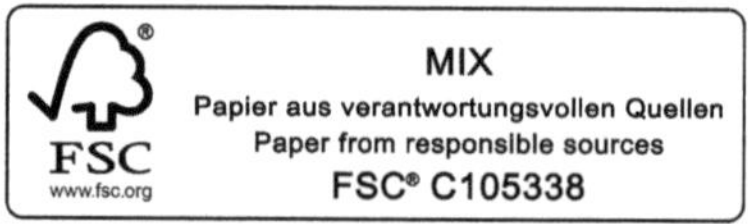

Printed by Books on Demand GmbH, Norderstedt / Germany